Biohacking Weight Loss for Beginners

A step by step guide on effortless weight loss and transforming your mind and body to a healthier you

Brittany Hills

Table of contents

Introduction

First of all,

"I wasn't sure I would make it. My health was fast declining, and my weight had become dangerously out of hand. In search of a way out, I dove into the realm of biohacking and came upon plenty of methods supported by science that changed my body and ultimately spared my life.

I give you access to these game-changing discoveries in "Biohacks for Weight Loss." This book is not a miracle drug or a fast-fix diet. It's a thorough manual for figuring out the biology of your body and maximizing it for long-term weight loss.

This is what you will discover:

The fundamental reasons behind weight gain and the strategies for resolving them.
- Biohacking methods to improve digestion, reduce cravings, and increase metabolism.
- How to maximize your ability to stop eating out of emotion and have a healthy connection with food.

One answer that works for everyone is not what this book is. Because everybody is different, what suits one individual could not suit another. Rather, consider this book as a toolbox full of methods and tools that you may try out to see what suits you the best.

We'll go into the exciting realm of biohacking for weight loss in the upcoming chapters, covering everything from improving your sleep quality to adjusting your food and everything in between. Prepare yourself to set out on a path to a more contented and healthy you."

Brief Overview of Biohacking for Weight Loss

Biohacking, also referred to as "human enhancement," encompasses everything from attempts to boost brain function to quicker weight loss, making small, gradual modifications to one's diet, lifestyle, and physique to enhance one's health and well-being. While some hacks can be tried safely at home and yield diverse effects, others may present health dangers.

Through a do-it-yourself (DIY) approach, biohacking is a type of human enhancement where individuals try to modify some components of their biology to boost their well-being, performance, or health. Certain forms of biohacking, like intermittent fasting, have been practiced for a long time.

Smartwatches are an example of technology-based biohacking devices that give users a plethora of bodily data, enabling them to make health and performance-related adjustments.

For a variety of reasons, people may choose to manipulate their biology, including to be in charge of their health and investigate fresh and alternative approaches, cure what they believe is amiss in an attempt to prolong their lives.

According to Brea Lofton, a registered dietitian, and nutritionist for health and wellness company Lumen, biohacking is the practice of using techniques derived from areas like genetics, biology, neuroscience, and nutrition to improve physical or mental performance, enhance overall health and well-being, or achieve a specific health outcome (like weight loss).

Dave Asprey, author of Smarter, Not Harder: The Biohacker's Guide to Getting the Body and Mind You Want describes biohacking as a global movement centered on the notion that you can alter both your internal and external surroundings to fully control your biology. He said at the 2023 annual Biohacking Conference in Orlando, Florida, that "control" for most individuals means wanting to be better, not merely alright.

According to him, hackers look at something they want to [access] and don't know what it is, so they just poke at it until it behaves the way they want. Then, they alter how they log in to take control of the system.

The concept essentially means that your health condition shouldn't be determined by chance, fate, or heredity. Rather, biohacking is the practice of manipulating one's neural system and physiology to achieve optimal, intelligent, and effective functioning.

The theory is that instead of using carbs as fuel, the body starts producing energy from fat. The term "keto" refers to a chemical that is produced by the body termed "ketone bodies." Body sculptors utilize this technique frequently to minimize their body fat percentage and for fat loss.

When you practice biohacking, you view your body as a system, with food serving as an input and vitality, energy, and mood serving as outputs. It may also encompass other objectives, such as losing weight.

To put it simply, we must track or evaluate specific aspects of our diet and lifestyle and pay attention to the effects on our bodies. You continuously adjust your food intake to get the desired results, based on your observations and your body's feelings.

Examples of Biohacking

Certain biohacking examples nowadays are so popular that they might be written off as normal aspects of daily existence. Others might appear more out of the ordinary and like trends of the future.

Boosters Known as "smart drugs," or nootropics, are a class of chemicals that are widely used in biohacking.

Nootropics that don't require a prescription can be found as tablets, beverages, and foods. They contain ingredients that might improve brain function. Caffeine and creatine are two examples.

Wearable technology that is worn Smartwatches, head-mounted displays, and fitness bands are examples of common wearable devices in today's world. They could be used by people to: monitor certain areas of their health and utilize the information to make adjustments, accomplish their health and fitness objectives monitor the cycles of reproductive health

The Various Forms of Biohacking

The practice of biohacking is not uniform. The three most common kinds are grinders, nutrigenomics, and DIY biology.

DIY biohacking, often known as garage biology, is the practice of scientific specialists imparting knowledge and biohacking techniques to non-experts in scientific domains.

This makes it possible for more people to experiment on themselves outside of restricted settings. DIY biology encompasses several biohacking domains, such as nutrition and microbiology, and Synthesis and medical biology

Nutrigenomics is an area of biohacking that focuses on the genetic interactions between food and individuals. It also looks at how a person's genes impact how their body reacts to certain foods.

Biohackers who identify as grinders see themselves as the originators of human enhancement. This kind of biohacking typically involves under-the-skin implants and the use of technology for physical adjustments.

Understanding Your Body

The relative proportions of the various body parts—most notably, lean mass and fat mass—are referred to as body composition. It offers a more thorough and precise picture of our physical composition than just body weight calculations.

Understanding the distribution of fat and muscle in our bodies is essential when assessing our general health and well-being, and this can be done by looking at our body composition.

Knowing the difference between lean and fat mass is crucial to understanding body composition. The quantity of body fat or adipose tissue that makes up our bodies is referred to as fat mass.

Although a certain quantity of body fat is required for energy storage, hormone regulation, and insulation, an excessive buildup of fat can have negative health implications.

On the other hand, lean mass includes everything including connective tissues, muscles, bones, and organs that are not fat. Supporting metabolism, physical strength, and general functionality are all greatly aided by lean mass.

One cannot stress how important it is to keep a good body composition. Gaining too much weight, especially in the visceral area, has been associated with an increased risk of heart disease, type 2 diabetes, stroke, and several cancers. Furthermore, being overweight can cause stress on joints and raise the risk of musculoskeletal issues.

Furthermore, a greater percentage of lean mass is linked to better insulin sensitivity, better metabolic health, and a lower risk of chronic illnesses. It offers a strong basis for overall vitality, mobility, and physical performance. Achieving and preserving a healthy body composition improves our overall health and well-being in addition to our outer looks.

Determining your body composition is more important than just using your weight as a health indicator. We may monitor our progress throughout weight loss or muscle building efforts, better understand our specific health risks, and make educated judgments about our exercise and nutrition regimens by determining the ratio of fat mass to lean mass.

We will delve into the idea of biohacking and how it may be used to optimise body composition in the upcoming parts. We can deliberately target fat loss while maintaining and enhancing lean mass by utilising biohacking techniques, opening the door to a stronger, healthier body.

Nutritional Biohacks

A key component of fat loss is nutrition, and biohacking provides cutting-edge methods to maximize this part of our trip.

The science that studies the interactions between food and genes is called nutrigenomics. The theory underlying this diet biohacking is that by comprehending the various ways in which foods impact our health, we may map out our body's entire genetic expression.

We may then use this mapping to determine the best eating plan for ourselves. It also provides us with a window into how various nutrients affect our emotions, ideas, and actions.

Many biohacking instances (genetically engineered implants, neurohacking technology, and the like) border on the strange, and some call for making more sensible and organic dietary adjustments. Let's look at a few innovative dietary biohacks that are popular in the fat loss community.

The Keto Diet

The ability of the ketogenic diet to encourage quick fat loss without sacrificing muscle mass has made it more well-liked. The goal of this high-fat, low-carb diet is to put the body into a state of ketosis, where it uses fat as its main energy source rather than glucose. Through a dramatic reduction in carbohydrates and an increase in healthy fat consumption, the ketogenic diet stimulates the body to burn fat that has been stored as fuel.

The ketogenic diet has several advantages, such as increased insulin sensitivity, decreased hunger, and better fat burning. The results of fat metabolism during ketosis, known as ketones, offer a consistent supply of energy to the muscles and brain. This metabolic state can result in better blood sugar regulation, more satiety, and effective fat loss.

Intermittent Fasting (IF)
IF is a cyclical eating pattern in which there are intervals of eating and fasting.

Different fasting procedures exist, such as 16/8 (fasting for 16 hours and eating within an 8-hour window), 5:2 (eating regularly for 5 days then drastically cutting calories for 2 non-consecutive days), and alternate-day fasting.

IF provides several ways to encourage fat loss. The body starts metabolizing stored fat for energy during the fasting period while its glycogen stores are being depleted.

This encourages the burning of fat and helps create a calorie deficit. Furthermore, IF may enhance hormone balance, cellular repair, and metabolic flexibility, promoting total fat loss and metabolic health.

Personalized Nutrition
Genetic testing has provided new information about how our distinct genetic composition affects how we react to certain foods and nutrients.

Using this data, personalized nutrition creates meal planning and dietary guidelines specific to a person's genetic profile.

Personalized diets can maximize fat reduction results by detecting genetic variants associated with metabolism, appetite management, and nutritional absorption.

It assists in determining the best macronutrient ratios, dietary selections, and times for a particular person to maximize fat reduction and advance general health.

To further tailor dietary recommendations, personalized nutrition also takes into account variables including food intolerances, sensitivities, and allergies.

Combining genetic testing with customized diet programs can enable people to maximize their fat-loss efforts according to their unique genetic makeup.

By avoiding the trial-and-error process that general diet plans frequently entail, this precise method helps increase the likelihood of long-term fat loss and healthier body composition.

Optimizing your body composition can be made more interesting by implementing these nutritional biohacks into your fat reduction plan.

Before making any significant dietary changes, you should, however, speak with medical specialists or trained dietitians, particularly if you have any dietary limitations or pre-existing medical concerns.

Recall that biohacking strategies are designed to be individualized and specific to your requirements, helping you to reach your weight loss objectives in a long-lasting and efficient way.

Biohacking Exercise

Exercise is a great way to improve body composition and maximize fat loss. Exercise methods that surpass conventional methods are introduced by biohacking. Let's look at some innovative exercise biohacks that can completely transform your approach to losing weight.

High-intensity interval training, or HIIT, is a type of exercise that alternates short bursts of vigorous activity with rest intervals. This method improves cardiovascular fitness and encourages fat reduction by taxing the anaerobic and aerobic systems. Human growth hormone (HGH) is produced at a higher level during high-intensity interval training (HIIT) and is involved in both muscle growth and fat metabolism.

The capacity of HIIT to raise heart rate and maintain it there after a workout is over is the science behind it. The term "afterburn effect" or excess post-exercise oxygen consumption (EPOC) refers to this phenomenon. HIIT exercises increase EPOC, which results in sustained fat oxidation and calorie burning for hours following the activity.

You can incorporate high-intensity interval training (HIIT) into your workout regimen by doing bodyweight exercises, cycling, or sprinting. Because of its adaptability and effectiveness, HIIT is a time-efficient and successful fat-loss method.

Resistance Training:

Although aerobic workouts have long been the focus for fat loss, weightlifting, sometimes referred to as resistance training, is becoming more and more recognized for its profound effects on body composition.

Resistance training increases lean muscle mass, which aids in fat loss. Muscle burns more calories at rest than fat since it is a metabolically active type of tissue. People can increase their resting metabolic rate and burn more fat even when they aren't exercising via resistance training to gain and maintain muscle.

Another advantage of resistance training is developing a toned and shaped body. Reduction of fat leads to a more visually pleasing appearance and improved body composition as muscle definition increases.

Metabolic Conditioning:

Also referred to as MetCon, metabolic conditioning is a type of rigorous exercise that increases metabolism and improves fat burning by fusing components of strength and cardiovascular training. Compound movements are usually performed throughout these workouts with little to no recovery in between, making for an intense and metabolically demanding training session.

MetCon exercises can be performed in a variety of ways, including Tabata training, circuit training, and functional training. MetCon workouts improve cardiovascular fitness, raise heart rate, increase calorie burn, and promote fat reduction by combining multi-joint activities and minimizing rest periods.

MetCon workouts can benefit from innovative training techniques, such as the use of unusual equipment like battle ropes, kettlebells, or suspension trainers, which can increase workout diversity and intensity. These workouts are dynamic, which means they work a variety of muscle groups and increase the amount of energy and fat that is used.

You can get amazing results from your exercises and maximize your fat reduction program by incorporating these exercise biohacks. To guarantee correct form and safety during your workouts, don't forget to speak with a certified fitness expert or exercise specialist.

To prevent overdoing it or getting hurt, pay attention to your body and gradually increase the duration and intensity of your workouts. You can improve your body composition and fat reduction efforts by combining the best exercise biohacks.

Sleep Optimization

First of all, It is harder than ever to get the right amount of sleep in the fast-paced world of today.

Although sleep is frequently disregarded concerning weight loss, it is crucial for controlling hormone levels and metabolism.

Insufficient sleep has the potential to upset the hormonal equilibrium linked to appetite control, resulting in heightened cravings and reduced feelings of fullness. It may also reduce glucose metabolism and insulin sensitivity, which makes fat-burning less effective.

Recognizing the Value of Sleep:

A basic biological function, sleep is essential to preserving our mental, emotional, and physical health. Our bodies heal wounds, solidify memories, and control our emotions when we sleep. Inadequate sleep has been connected to numerous health problems, such as obesity, diabetes as well as heart problems.

Establishing the Ideal Ambience for Sleep:

Making an environment that is suitable to sleep is one of the most important steps in maximizing your sleep. This entails purchasing a cozy mattress and pillows and maintaining a cool, quiet, and dark bedroom. Limiting your exposure to screens and artificial light before bed is also recommended, as these can interfere with your body's normal circadian rhythm.

Creating a Sleep Schedule:

Your body can be told to slow down and get ready for sleep by establishing a nightly routine. This can involve engaging in relaxing activities like deep breathing exercises or meditation, as well as hobbies like reading a book or having a warm bath. Reducing coffee and stimulating activities in the hours before bed can also aid in improving sleep quality.

The Functions of Exercise and Diet:

Exercise and diet have a big impact on how well you sleep. Maintaining a healthy, balanced diet and getting regular exercise will help you sleep better overall by regulating your sleep-wake cycle. Preventing sleep disturbances can also be achieved by avoiding large meals and caffeine close to bedtime.

Controlling Anxiety and Stress:

Your ability to sleep can be significantly impacted by stress and anxiety. By engaging in stress-reduction practices like yoga, meditation, or mindfulness, you can relax and get better quality sleep. Additionally, if stress and anxiety are interfering with your sleep, it may be helpful to seek assistance from a mental health specialist.

In summary:

To improve the quality of your sleep, turn off electronics at least an hour before bed, keep your bedroom cold and dark, and use relaxing methods like reading or meditation.

Making sleep a priority and getting enough good sleep every night can help you maintain a healthy hormone balance, boost your energy, and achieve the best possible results with fat loss.

Improving your sleep quality is crucial for your general health and well-being. By putting the plans into practice you can get better sleep and wake up every day feeling invigorated and renewed.

Stress management

Introduction

Stress has become a regular companion for many in today's fast-paced society, often wreaking havoc on our health and well-being. Stress can be a significant obstacle to weight loss because it alters our metabolism, eating preferences, and level of desire in general. To assist your biohacking journey towards a healthy you, we will look deeper into the relationship between stress and weight increase in this chapter and examine practical stress management approaches.

The Link Between Stress and Weight Loss

Cortisol, a hormone that can stimulate hunger and cause fat storage, especially around the abdomen, is released when stress is experienced. Stress can also cause sleep disorders, increase appetites for foods heavy in fat and sugar, and decrease the desire to exercise. It may be difficult to reach your objectives and undermine your weight loss attempts due to all of these issues.

Comprehending Stress Reduction

Mindfulness Meditation: Each day, spend at least ten to fifteen minutes practicing mindfulness meditation. Take a comfortable seat, close your eyes, and concentrate on breathing. Bring your thoughts back to your breathing when they stray. You can enhance your connection with food, lower stress levels, and become more self-aware by engaging in this exercise.

Frequent Exercise: Exercise regularly to improve your mood and lower stress levels. Try to incorporate strength training, flexibility training, and cardiovascular activity into your routine. Make time for the things you enjoy doing daily.

Good Sleep: Try to get seven to nine hours of good sleep every night. Establish a calming nighttime routine, avoid using electronics right before bed, and make sure your sleeping space is comfortable for sound sleep. Good sleep can help with weight loss and lower stress levels.

Relaxation Techniques: To lower stress, include relaxation techniques in your everyday activities. Try yoga, progressive muscular relaxation, or deep breathing techniques. These methods can ease your body and mind, allowing you to manage stress more easily.

Good Eating Practices: Keep a diet full of fruits, vegetables, whole grains, lean meats, and other nutrients. Steer clear of excessive alcohol, coffee, and sugary food intake as they might increase stress levels. Stress reduction and blood sugar stabilization can both be achieved by eating regular, wholesome meals.

Social Support: To get emotional support, and maintain relationships with friends and family. Talk to people about your struggles and achievements, and get expert assistance if necessary. You can handle stress better if you have a solid support system.

Establishing Objectives: Establish attainable and reasonable objectives for your weight loss journey. Divide more ambitious objectives into more doable segments, and acknowledge and appreciate your progress along the way. This might boost your drive for success and lessen overwhelming feelings.

Conclusion

Effective stress management is crucial to a weight loss program that works. You can lessen tension, assist your biohacking endeavors, and reach your weight loss objectives by implementing these doable actions into your everyday routine. Recall that development requires time, so as you begin your journey, practice patience and self-care

Enhancements and Biohacking

Supplementing with additional assistance to optimize metabolism, accelerate fat burning, and improve overall body composition can be a useful strategy for biohacking fat reduction. It is imperative, therefore, to handle supplements cautiously and under a doctor's supervision.

Let's examine how supplements can biohack fat loss and some cutting-edge solutions to think about.

Synopsis of Supplements:
Products called supplements are made to support a balanced diet and way of life.

They include particular nutrients, herbal extracts, or bioactive chemicals and are available in a variety of formats, such as capsules, powders, liquids, or gummies.

Supplements support metabolic function, optimize body composition, and help the body's natural fat-burning activities when taken as directed.

It's crucial to remember that using supplements won't help you lose weight faster or substitute for a healthy diet. They should be used in addition to a healthy lifestyle that consists of frequent exercise and a balanced diet.

Supplements for Burning Fat:
Supplements that burn fat are made to boost and improve fat metabolism, encouraging increased calorie expenditure and fat burning.

These supplements frequently include substances that have been linked to increased thermogenesis—the body's production of heat—and fat oxidation, such as caffeine, green tea extract, forskolin, or synephrine.

Thermogenic supplements function by boosting energy expenditure, raising metabolic rate, and activating the central nervous system. They may give people a little energy boost and assist them in breaking through weight reduction plateaus.

Natural Compounds: A few natural compounds have drawn interest for their ability to improve fat reduction in addition to manufactured fat-burning supplements. These substances include conjugated linoleic acid (CLA), capsaicin (found in chili peppers), forskolin, and green tea extract.

Catechins, which are found in green tea extract, have been demonstrated to accelerate metabolism and improve fat oxidation. The plant forskolin, which comes from the Coleus forskohlii plant, may help with fat loss by raising adenylate cyclase levels, which trigger the body's mechanisms that burn fat.

It has been discovered that capsaicin, the substance that gives chili peppers their fiery flavor, increases thermogenesis and encourages fat burning. A fatty acid called CLA, which is present in meat and dairy products, may aid in improving body composition and lowering body fat.

It's crucial to remember that although these organic substances appear promising, each person may respond differently to them in terms of efficacy. Moreover, their effect on weight loss should be considered in the context of a holistic strategy that incorporates healthy eating, regular exercise, and lifestyle adjustments.

Consulting a Healthcare Professional: It's important to speak with a licensed healthcare provider or certified dietician before adding any supplements to your fat reduction program. They can determine your specific requirements, consider any drug interactions or pre-existing conditions, and offer advice on how to take supplements responsibly.

Since supplementation is very personalized, what is effective for one person might not be for another. A medical expert can assist in determining any underlying nutritional imbalances or inadequacies and suggest certain supplements that are in line with your objectives and general well-being.

Always take caution when using supplements, and combine them with other lifestyle changes such as eating a balanced diet and getting regular exercise.

Stress the value of whole foods and concentrate on making the best possible dietary and lifestyle choices before thinking of using supplements as a fat-loss biohacking technique.

You can maximize the potential benefits of supplements by using them sensibly and wisely, putting your general health and well-being first.

Biofeedback and Tracking

With the help of a technique called biofeedback, people can learn to take control of their body's natural processes, such as heart rate, blood pressure, muscular tension, and skin temperature, and so enhance their health.

Biofeedback and tracking are essential components of biohacking, allowing individuals to monitor and adjust their body's responses for optimal health and performance. This chapter explores the definition, types, integration into biohacking, home practices, benefits, and practical tips for effective implementation.

What is Biofeedback?
Biofeedback is a process that enables individuals to learn how to control physiological functions such as heart rate, muscle tension, and brainwave activity. It involves using sensors to monitor these bodily functions and providing real-time feedback, allowing individuals to make conscious adjustments.

Types of Biofeedback
1. Electromyography (EMG): Measures muscle activity and tension.

2. Electroencephalography (EEG): Monitors brainwave activity.
3. Galvanic Skin Response (GSR): Tracks changes in skin conductance, often related to stress levels.
4. Heart Rate Variability (HRV): Measures the variation in time intervals between heartbeats, reflecting autonomic nervous system activity.

Biofeedback in Biohacking

Biofeedback plays a crucial role in biohacking by providing valuable insights into how our bodies respond to various stimuli. By utilizing biofeedback data, biohackers can tailor their diet, exercise, and lifestyle choices to optimize their health and performance.

Practicing Biofeedback at Home

While professional biofeedback sessions are available, there are also ways to practice biofeedback at home:

- Wearable Devices: Use wearable devices that track metrics such as heart rate, sleep patterns, and activity levels.
- Mobile Apps: Utilize mobile apps that provide biofeedback training and allow you to track your progress over time.

- Mindfulness and Meditation: Practice mindfulness and meditation techniques to improve your ability to control physiological responses.

 Benefits of Biofeedback
- Stress Reduction: Biofeedback can help individuals manage stress by providing real-time feedback on stress levels and teaching relaxation techniques.
- Performance Enhancement: Athletes can use biofeedback to improve their performance by optimizing their physiological responses during training and competition.
- Health Optimization: Biofeedback can be used to improve overall health by identifying and addressing imbalances in the body.

Practical Tips for Biofeedback and Tracking
1. Consistency: Regular practice is key to seeing meaningful results from biofeedback.
2. Setting Goals: Establish clear goals for your biofeedback practice to track progress and stay motivated.
3. Seek Professional Guidance: Consider working with a biofeedback therapist or healthcare provider to ensure safe and effective practice.

In conclusion, biofeedback and tracking are powerful tools in the biohacking toolkit, offering valuable insights into our body's responses and enabling us to optimize our health and performance. By integrating biofeedback into our daily lives and practicing mindfulness, we can unlock our full potential for health and well-being.

Personalized Approaches

Unlocking Your Body's Potential

Imagine embarking on a weight loss journey where every step is specifically designed for you, considering your unique genetic makeup, nutritional requirements, and lifestyle choices.

This chapter delves into the personalized approach of biohacking, revealing how to optimize your body's potential for shedding those unwanted pounds.

Understanding Your Body's Blueprint

Before diving into any weight loss regimen, it's crucial to understand your body's blueprint. This involves analyzing your genetic predispositions, metabolism, and any underlying health conditions.

Tools like genetic testing and comprehensive health assessments can provide valuable insights into how your body functions and metabolizes nutrients.

Tailoring Your Nutrition Plan

When it comes to nutrition, there is no one size fits all. Biohacking emphasizes the importance of customizing your diet based on your individual needs and preferences.

Start by identifying foods that fuel your body and eliminate those that hinder your progress. Experiment with different macronutrient ratios, meal timing, and portion sizes to find what works best for you.

Monitoring Your Body's Responses

Tracking your progress is essential for fine-tuning your weight loss journey. Utilize wearable devices, and apps, or simply keep a journal to monitor metrics such as weight, body composition, energy levels, and mood.

Pay attention to how your body responds to different foods, exercises, and lifestyle changes, and adjust accordingly.

Harnessing the Power of Mindfulness

Weight loss isn't just about what you eat; it's also about how you eat. Mindful eating should be practiced by taking your time to savor each bite, getting in tune with signals from your body like your body's hunger and fullness cues, and avoiding distractions during meals.

Cultivate a positive mindset by focusing on progress rather than perfection and celebrating small victories along the way.

Implementing Strategic Exercise

Exercise is a key component of any weight loss plan, but not all workouts are created equal. Choose activities that you enjoy and that align with your goals and physical abilities.

Incorporate a combination of cardiovascular, strength training, and flexibility exercises to maximize fat burning and muscle building.

Fine-Tuning Your Lifestyle Habits

Your daily habits play a significant role in your weight loss success. Optimize your sleep quality and quantity to support hormone regulation and metabolism.

Manage stress through techniques such as meditation, deep breathing, or engaging in hobbies that bring you joy. Surround yourself with a supportive environment that encourages healthy choices and accountability.

Real-Life Examples and Practical Tips

To illustrate the personalized approach of biohacking for weight loss, let's consider a hypothetical case study:

Sarah, a 35-year-old working mother with a family history of obesity, decides to embark on a biohacking journey to lose weight and improve her overall health. After conducting a genetic analysis, she discovers that she has a predisposition to insulin resistance and benefits from a low-carbohydrate diet.

Sarah crafts a nutrition plan focused on whole foods rich in protein, healthy fats, and fiber while minimizing refined sugars and processed carbs. She experiments with intermittent fasting and finds that it helps regulate her blood sugar levels and curb cravings.

Using a fitness tracker, Sarah monitors her daily steps and sets achievable goals to increase her physical activity gradually. She incorporates high-intensity interval training (HIIT) workouts into her routine, which she can do at home to accommodate her busy schedule.

Mindful eating practices help Sarah become more attuned to her body's hunger and fullness signals, preventing mindless snacking and emotional eating. She practices stress management techniques such as yoga and journaling to cope with the demands of her job and family responsibilities.

Over time, Sarah's personalized approach to biohacking yields impressive results. Not only does she lose weight, but she also experiences improvements in her energy levels, mood, and overall well-being.

In Conclusion

The personalized approach of biohacking empowers individuals to take control of their weight loss journey by understanding and optimizing their body's unique needs. By tailoring nutrition, monitoring body responses, practicing mindfulness, implementing strategic exercise, and fine-tuning lifestyle habits, anyone can achieve lasting results and unlock their body's full potential.

Potential Challenges and Solutions

Embarking on a biohacking journey for weight loss can be incredibly rewarding, but it's not without its challenges. In this chapter, we'll explore some common hurdles faced by individuals undertaking this transformative journey and provide practical solutions to overcome them.

Challenge 1: Initial Resistance to Change

Description: Many people find it challenging to adopt new habits and make significant lifestyle changes, especially when it comes to diet and exercise.

Solution:
1. Start Slowly: Gradually introduce changes into your routine to allow for adjustment without feeling overwhelmed.
2. **Set Realistic Goals**: Break down your weight loss goals into smaller, achievable milestones to keep yourself motivated.
3. Find Support: Surround yourself with a supportive community of friends, family, or fellow biohackers who can offer encouragement and accountability.

Challenge 2: Plateaus and Stagnation

Description: It's common to experience plateaus or periods of stagnation in weight loss progress, where the scale refuses to budge despite your efforts.

Solution:
1. **Reassess Your Approach**: Take a step back and evaluate your current biohacking strategies. Are there any areas where you can make adjustments or improvements?
2. **Mix Up Your Routine**: Introduce variety into your diet and exercise regimen to prevent boredom and keep your body guessing.
3. **Focus on Non-Scale Victories**: Shift your focus away from the number on the scale and celebrate other victories, such as increased energy levels or improved mood.

Challenge 3: Emotional Eating and Cravings

Description: Emotional eating and cravings can derail even the most well-intentioned weight loss efforts, leading to overeating and potential setbacks.

Solution:

1. Identify Triggers: Pay attention to the emotions or situations that trigger your cravings, and develop alternative coping mechanisms such as journaling or deep breathing exercises.
2. Practice Mindful Eating: Slow down and savor each bite, paying attention to hunger and fullness cues rather than mindlessly consuming food.
3. Stock Up on Healthy Options: Keep your kitchen stocked with nutritious, satisfying snacks to curb cravings and prevent impulse eating.

Challenge 4: Lack of Time and Resources

Description: Busy schedules and limited resources can make it challenging to prioritize healthy habits and maintain consistency in your biohacking journey.

Solution:
1. Plan Ahead: Take time to meal prep and plan your workouts to maximize efficiency and minimize decision fatigue.
2. Make Use of Technology: Utilize apps, online resources, and wearable devices to streamline tracking and monitoring of your progress.

3. Focus on Quality Over Quantity: Quality of exercise and nutrition is more important than quantity. Focus on making the most of the time and resources you have available.

Challenge 5: Social Pressure and Peer Influence

Description: Social situations and peer pressure can make it difficult to stick to your biohacking goals, especially when faced with temptation from friends or family.

Solution:
1. Communicate Your Goals: Be open and honest with your loved ones about your weight loss journey and ask for their support in helping you stay on track.
2. Find Healthy Alternatives: Suggest alternative activities or venues for social gatherings that align with your goals, such as going for a hike instead of meeting for drinks.
3. Lead by Example: Set a positive example for those around you by demonstrating healthy habits and showing that prioritizing your health is important to you.

In conclusion, while the path to weight loss through biohacking may present its challenges, with determination, perseverance, and the right strategies in place, you can overcome these obstacles and achieve lasting success in your journey toward a healthier, happier you.

Ethical Considerations

Ethics play a crucial role in any health-related endeavor, including biohacking for weight loss. In this chapter, we'll explore some of the key ethical considerations to keep in mind as you embark on your biohacking journey.

Respect for Autonomy

Explanation: Autonomy refers to the right of individuals to make their own decisions about their health and well-being.

Application: Ensure that any biohacking practices you engage in are based on your own informed choices and align with your values and beliefs.

Beneficence and Non-Maleficence

Explanation: Beneficence refers to the duty to promote the well-being of others, while non-maleficence refers to the duty to not harm.

Application: When biohacking for weight loss, prioritize practices that are beneficial to your health and well-being while avoiding those that may cause harm or have negative side effects.

Justice and Fairness

Explanation: Justice involves treating individuals fairly and ensuring that everyone has equal access to health-promoting opportunities.

Application: Be mindful of the resources you use in your biohacking journey, and consider how your actions may impact others.

Conclusion

In this book, we've explored the transformative power of biohacking in achieving your weight loss goals and optimizing your health. Throughout this book, we've delved into the science behind biohacking, practical strategies for implementation, and ethical considerations to keep in mind.

We've learned that biohacking is not just about losing weight; it's about understanding your body, optimizing your health, and embracing a holistic approach to wellness. By harnessing the power of personalized nutrition, targeted exercise, and mindful living, you can unlock your body's full potential and achieve lasting results.

As you embark on your biohacking journey, remember that progress is not always linear. There may be challenges and setbacks along the way, but each step forward is a step closer to your goals. Stay committed to your health and well-being, and be patient with yourself as you navigate this path.

I encourage you to continue your exploration of biohacking and wellness beyond this book.

Seek out additional resources, connect with like-minded individuals, and continue to educate yourself on the latest advancements in health and wellness.

Above all, remember that your health is your greatest asset. Embrace your journey to health and wellness with enthusiasm and determination.

The power to transform your life starting today, is in your hands